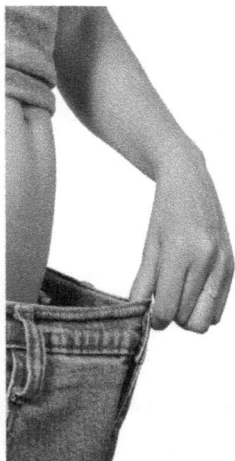

THE 5-HOUR DIET!

TURN YOUR BODY INTO A FAT-BURNING MACHINE!

T.J. ROHLEDER

Take a Guru to Lunch
P.O. Box 198
Goessel, Kansas 67053

ISBN 1-933356-57-X

<u>INTRODUCTION</u>

This small book can change your life. It can help you...

- Lose all the weight you want.

- Look and feel better.

- Have more energy and vitality.

- Sleep better.

- And even live longer!

That's a tall order. I know. But keep an open mind and read closely.

By the time you're done going through this small book, you'll have all the secrets you need to turn your body into a fat-burning furnace.

Does that sound like hype? Well, it's not! I'm proof.

This 5-Hour Diet will turn up the volume on your metabolism and help you to lose the weight you want to lose, and so much more. So don't let the size of this small book fool you. It's a small book that can produce big results when you use the fat-burning secrets I'm about to share with you.

With all that said, let's begin...

Oh – one more thing... If you like this little book, download the Audio Book version from Audible.com – and listen to this book in its original 40-minute audio interview format. Listening and reading this book might give you the ultimate motivation to start the 5-Hour Diet and change your life.

CHAPTER ONE

What is the 5-Hour Diet? And How Does It Work?

This diet will change your life.

I know that sounds dramatic, but it has changed my life and added years to it. It's a diet that's given me more energy, makes me feel better, and it's helped me lose and maintain my weight.

This weight was getting harder to lose as I got older, and it felt so good to lose it.

Thanks to this diet, I'm 63 years old and still have the same weight I had in high school. That's important to me because it becomes harder to lose and maintain weight as we get older.

This diet is simple to understand and easy to use. It's called Intermittent Fasting. You can find a ton of stuff online about it. The 5-Hour Diet is a unique way to practice this diet.

My friend, Jay, may have saved my life (or added years to my life) when he told me about this diet. Before this, I had tried all kinds of crazy diets, but Intermittent Fasting is different because it's based on this premise...

It's not what you eat;
it's when you eat.

With this diet, you go through a significant daily period where you're not eating. You already do this when you're sleeping. So, if you sleep 8 hours a day, you're not consuming any calories during those hours. And if you're like most people, you're not hungry when they wake up. So going 10 to 12 hours without any calories is easy. Intermittent Fasting means you stretch that period for as long as you can.

I call this the 5-Hour Diet because of my unique perspective on Intermittent Fasting. I can't wait to share this with you! Not only can this change your life, but I'm convinced it can save your life and add years to your life, add life to your years!

This diet will give you more energy and vitality. It changes your metabolism and turns your body into a fat-burning machine!   I know that sounds like hype. Still, I call it the 5-Hour Diet because I realized, having been on this diet for a couple of years and have experimented with different ways of doing it. The most important lesson I've learned is that the key to making this diet an essential part of your life is to learn how to deal with the short periods of hunger you'll go through every day.

This is the only challenge that you must learn how to overcome. That's the purpose of this small book and the audio recording on which it is based.

If you can learn how to live with

these small doses of daily pain, you can lose weight fast, live longer, and eat whatever you want. I'll help you make it easy. And this is proven to work. It's as simple as learning how to get through the 3 to 5 hours a day when you're experiencing a little hunger.

The idea behind this diet came from my friend, Jay.

Jay is the man who got me excited about this diet. Like me, he's been trying to maintain and lose weight for years. He's also tried all the various diets. Most have left him frustrated. But this diet is different because it's focused on when you eat and not what you eat. I was having a conversation with Jay about this diet, and I said, 'The whole trick to this diet is your ability to deal with a little pain or hunger every day. "If you can do that, you can master this diet."

The title for this book came from a conversation with Jay. He's the friend who got me on this diet. Jay and I have both tried many different diets; like most people trying to lose weight or maintain weight, you try everything. And I realized that the only real problem with this diet is, or the only obstacle, if you will, the only challenge, that's another good way of saying it, you must be willing to just put up with a bit of hunger every day.

Most people have never really been hungry. You'll hear them saying things like you learn how to live with it and even embrace it. I'll give you some of my best tips, tricks, and strategies to do this.

In summary, if you can get through those 3 to 5 hours a day (and you can!), then you can master this diet and change your life. It's that simple. And with enough practice, it's that easy. Get good at dealing with this hunger (which I will help you do), and you will turn your body into a fat-burning machine.

And that brings us to the next question..

CHAPTER TWO

Can You Eat Whatever You Want and Still Lose Weight?

With this diet, you are limiting the calories that you put in your body every day. Study after study shows that one of the big secrets to longevity is to limit the calories that you consume each day. All diets try to achieve this. You are watching what you eat and trying to limit your calories.

My dad used to call salad rabbit food. He struggled with his weight all of his life, and he died before he had to die. He was 74 years old when he died. I am convinced that he could have easily added a decade or two onto his life if he would have just been on a diet that instead of eating all the time like he did, if he would have just gone a significant period of time.

Some people are on what they call a 20:4 Diet, where 4 hours a day they eat, they call it eating windows. I never liked that concept. I like the concept of starving windows. If you can just go through a period of 3 to 5 hours where you are hungry but you do not eat. I will show you some tips, tricks, and strategies. You can eat whatever you want, but most people try to eat a bunch of food. Cabbage soup diet is famous diet. I can't think of anything to give me more pleasure than that. You just eat salad, fruit, or you try to eat popcorn. There is all this low-calories, it's not doable, it's drudgery.

I am miserable on those diets. There is a little bit of misery, because that is why we call it the 5-Hour Diet. Most days I am hungry for about 3 hours. I could have called this the 3-Hour Diet instead of the 5 hours. However, there are some days when you are feeling a little bit of hunger for 3 to 5 hours. Get past those difficult periods, now you really can eat whatever you want. Because your stomach shrinks when you get on this diet, so naturally you can't eat as much. I start eating every day at 12:30 PM or 1:00 PM. I would like to eat huge meal, but I can't because my stomach actually shrinks. However, I do eat whatever I want, but I try to be sensible and get the amount of protein and nutrients that I needed. It's not just an all ice cream diet, that would not be healthy to just eat ice cream, cake, and cookies. However, every day I do have a sweet tooth.

I don't want to deprive myself from the foods that I enjoy i;e. Pizza, tacos, etc. I make sure that every day I have it. So, all of these diets where you just eat a bunch of celery or carrots that is torture.

Why torture yourself?

We call this the 5-Hour Diet because there is that period every day when you are somewhat torturing yourself a little bit. The pain of self-discipline is what I would call it.

You can eat whatever you want.

You can eat pizza, pasta, cake, and cookies because you don't want to eat as much, essentially you're eating two small meals a day, there is that window of time when you're eating versus the rest of the time when you're not taking any calories.

Naturally, you want to have some healthy food there too. You are more aware of food, but here is the point; food loses its power over you. When you are constantly shoving food in your face, there is that you do tend to feel hungry all the time. However, you are also eating because you are bored; you have never disciplined your body to do anything other than that.

Ultimately, food has more power and control over you than it should have. When you are on a diet like the 5-Hour Diet, the food really does lose its power over you.

In summary, you can eat all that stuff because your body now becomes more sensitive to that. Therefore, naturally I don't want to eat just carrots, salad, celery, and all of that either.

<u>CHAPTER THREE</u>

It's Called the 5-Hour Diet Because You are Focusing on the 3 to 5 Hours a Day When You are Feeling Hungry. That Magic Time Turns Your Body into a Fat-Burning Furnace.

I equate it with the way an athlete goes to the gym. When you talk to athletes, they interpret pain differently. Look at a long-distance runner, where they put their body through all kinds of the worst pain that I can even imagine. Some of them are crawling over the finish line. Some of them don't make it over the finish line on those long ultra-marathon runs of 50 to 100 miles through all kinds of rugged terrain. They have ambulances standing by, doctors are right there to save their lives. These people have a different way of defining what the word pain really means. This diet, I call it the 5-Hour Diet because it came from a conversation with the man who introduced me to this diet, my good friend, Jay. He is struggling with this diet too; we are encouraging each other, which I would recommend it. When this diet starts working for you, share it with as many other people as you can and encourage them to try it.

If you can learn to live with a little hunger for 3 to 5 hours every day, then you got this diet whipped. What you need is a habit of restricting the calories. It's so simple. That's one of the promises that we made in the beginning, you're starting as late in the day as you can, and you stop eating as soon as you can. Then you are willing to feel that hunger for just a few hours a day, but you change the definition of that hunger. What does that pain really mean?

Therefore, when I feel that pain, which I do, I know that's where the magic is happening. Everybody is different, but eventually your metabolism does change and you start losing weight. You're changing the meaning of that pain, you're seeing the benefits.

Short-Term Pain, Long-Term Gain

Every person that goes to the gym, they struggle to get their exercising done, they are willingly enduring a little bit of pain for periods of time every day. I have always admired them.

I start eating about 1:00 PM every day and I stop eating about 7:00 PM at night. I give myself a little bit of leniency and a little bit of a break every now and then, we are not robots, but you're 18 hours of not eating and 6 hours of eating. I am only enduring about 3 hours of pain every day.

I try to stay busy during those 3 hours. I have learned to live with a little bit of pain. It is the pain of discipline. It is a short-term pain every day that changes your metabolism, turns your body into that fat-burning machine that sounds like hype. Our metabolism does change. We are finding meaning in that pain, just like all forms of self-discipline.

CHAPTER FOUR

Where Does This Diet Shine Over All Other Weight-Loss Options?

Most diets put all of their focus on what you eat. I am talking about the intermittent diet, its focuses on when you eat not what you eat. It would be the key foundation of the intermittent diet or intermittent fasting. What differentiates the 5-Hour Diet from all of that is we are putting all of the focus on the 3 to 5 hours a day when you feel the actual pain of hunger?

However, when I called it the 5-Hour Diet that is not exactly not true. It is more like the 2 or 3-Hour Diet. By calling it the 5-Hour Diet, we are giving ourselves the benefit of a doubt. Everybody is different. In the beginning, you might experience some real hunger for maybe up to 5 hours a day. However, whether it's 2 hours, 3 hours, or 5 hours, this diet puts the emphasis on that. This is the part everybody wants to avoid. People don't like to feel hungry. It is just a perspective.

I have already talked about ultra-marathon runners, they place positive value on the pain that they go through, they get off on it, and it makes them feel great. I was on the paleo diet for a long time, where all you eat is protein, or things that our ancestors would have eaten.

To me, that is torture; I would rather go through 3 to 5 hours a day of being in some kind of pain and just get it over with every day because if you can do that, you can do this diet. You will get all of the benefits we talked about before. You will lose weight, you will live longer, you can eat whatever you want, it's easy and proven. Self-discipline is ultimate form of control. Most control is external control. Somebody standing over your shoulder with a clipboard, people are making demands on you. That is a terrible kind of control, where outer forces are controlling you.

Internal control or self-control is the ultimate form of control because it is something that you are consciously subjecting yourself to. Therefore, what you have to do is you have to find a way. What you are talking about are 3 to 5 hours a day where you are feeling hungry. All of this came because of weight loss, and there is no question about it. This is the ultimate way to reduce the amount of calories, and it turns your body into a fat-burning furnace. It changes your metabolism.

Those 3 to 5 hours a day when you ae hungry, sometimes it's just 2 hours a day, when I am feeling that pain oh hunger, that's when all of the magic and the miracles are occurring. That is when your metabolism is being changed, you are turning things around a teaching your body how to start burning all of that, the eating up all of the fat. This is one of my greatest discoveries.

Find something that keeps you so busy that you will not think about your hunger. You are making a game out of it, you are having fun with it, and you are creating those positive meanings in your pain. You just have to find or create various ways, because different things work at different times for different people. It is the easiest thing in the world. In fact, one of the real benefits of this diet, other than weight loss, you can sleep so much better on this diet.

Getting a good night's sleep is important, as you get older. There is nothing like a good night's sleep. You have to experiment. However, those 3 to 5 hours of hunger is that your mind is sharper, you think better, you have more energy. Sometimes, the energy comes and goes. This is the period of time when you are changing your metabolism; it's when all of the magic happens.

Turn your body into a
fat-burning machine

Here is one last idea. This idea is contrary to everything. Yet, you might want to experiment with this one too a little bit. Remember, I try to stay as busy as I can, get my mind off the fact that I am hungry. However, sometimes, I do the exact opposite. I just feel the pain of hunger, and this has been a very positive thing for me because I will just speak for myself, I did not even realize this until I got on this diet. However, most people are afraid of being hungry.

The last thing anybody wants is to live a life of complete torture, where you are measuring your meals out.

Although, I know the benefits from a health standpoint only. You are giving your digestive system a break. There is so much of your energy is being completely devoted to digesting the food you eat, and when you are eating food constantly, your body never gets a break, your metabolism is always working overtime. By having periods, whether it's 18 hours, again my prime target is every day to try to get as close to 1:00 PM in the afternoon before I eat anything.

I am drinking black coffee in the morning with no sugar, creamer, so there is no calories. There are benefits to fasting; people have known that for thousands of years. This gives you many of those same long-term health advantages.

People have been fasting for spiritual reasons. When your body is just not so busy, digesting that food, a lot of energy, it does change your energy.

CHAPTER FIVE

Final Words to Wrap This Up.

As you get older, the things that kept you things when you were young, your metabolism does change. Jay is interested in weight loss; I am interested in weight management more than weight loss. It is not as easy to stay thin anymore. I never heard about intermittent fasting until Jay told me about it. I really believe this has changed my life, as well as it will change your life. So share this with other people, get them on this diet. It can start being just a 12:12 diet. Most people can do that.

They can stop eating sooner at night and not just snack. The worst thing you can do is take a meal before you go to bed. That is a recipe for disease and sickness; it's just the worst thing you can do.

Stop eating as soon as you can
every night, start eating as late
as you can in the morning.

Go 12 by 12, 12 hours of just no
calories at all, and then try to expand it,
make a game out of it, but share it with
other. Life is meant to be shared.
Happiness is only real when it is shared.
The 12-step programs, which I have been
around for decades now, because of some
substance abuse issue I had in my earlier
life, it is all about sharing it with others. As
long as you are doing it sincerely, then you
are definitely benefited.

When you really do feel hungry,
watch your metabolism change over a quick
period because that is the whole benefits of
the turning your body into a fat-burning
furnace. This is a proven diet. It is easy to
do. It beats all other diets where you have to
eat foods that you don't want to eat and you
have to do things like counting the portions.
That naturally occurs on this diet. When

you are feeling some pain or discomfort, you
are not going to die here.

It is a **"Short-term pain for long-
term gain"**. Share it with other people.
This is the key to living longer. You are
never going to know that for a fact, but
life to your years. Hope you have
benefited from this diet.

<u>PROLOGUE</u>

Thank you for reading The 5-Hour Diet. Be sure to check out the audio book on Audible.com. This book is a written transcript of an audio conversation. Take a Guru to Lunch was founded on the premise that we were having a conversation over lunch. But in order for this to be a real conversation, you need to add your comments. Please reach out through our support desk and let me know what you think. Connect through tickets@heytj.com and mention "The 5-Hour Diet" in the subject line. Because I want to have a real conversation with you, I personally answer all messages. I look forward to hearing from you soon.